Home Remedies
For Heart Attack
And Strokes

Home Remedies
For Heart Attack
And Strokes

By Monica Sidoine,
S.N.H.S. Dip. Herbalism

DISCLAIMER

This book is to serve as an informational guide for use in the home. The remedies and procedures contained in this book are meant to supplement and are not intended to be a substitute for professional medical care. Please seek a qualified medical practitioner for all ailments. The author nor distributors takes no responsibility for customers choosing to treat themselves. Your use of this information is at your own risk.

ISBN - 13: 978-1534761308
ISBN - 10: 1534761306

Proof Read by Jasmine Ned Anunda

Printed By Create Space Publishing
United States of America

ACKNOWLEDGMENTS

I would like to thank all those who have contributed in one way or another to the completion of HOME REMEDIES FOR HEART ATTACK AND STROKES.

I thank God for giving me the vision, wisdom and good health to write this book. For all he has done and will continue to do in my life.

For the many prayer warriors who interceded on behalf of this project and also their moral support.

I thank my daughter Jasmine Ned Anunda for proof reading.

Thank you all.

Monica Sidoine.

PREFACE

The procedures in this Book was designed to be as simple as possible so that anyone will be able to follow them. Most of the items used are local things which you would either have at home, in your kitchen garden or can be easily purchased from the local market or health store for a very low cost.

TABLE OF CONTENTS

HEART ATTACK

What is a heart attack?
A heart attack is a sudden, serious, painful, and sometimes fatal interruption of the heart's normal functioning, especially due to a blockage in the coronary artery.

What are some of the signs?
Sudden chest pain, discomfort in upper body parts, shortness of breath, difficulty in breathing, changes in the pulse rate, dizziness, cold sweat, edema.

Other possible warning signs of a heart attack include: -
Feeling tired for no reason, nausea, vomiting, restlessness, intense anxiety, a fear of death, and a general feeling of being unwell.

What are the risk factors?
Aging, smoking, abnormal blood levels of certain lipids, diabetes, high blood pressure, lack of physical activity, obesity, chronic kidney disease, excessive alcohol consumption, the use of cocaine and amphetamines.

NATURAL REMEDIES

- Steep 1 teaspoon of cayenne powder to 1 cup of boiling water. Take ½oz doses or 2 capsules 3 times daily.
  N.B. Very excessive use can damage the kidneys.

- Steep 1oz of corn hairs to 1 liter of boiling water for 30 minutes.
  Drink 4 cups daily but not at night.

- Steep sesame seeds for 20 minutes. Strain and toast lightly. Take two teaspoons after breakfast and lunch.

- Steep 1oz of ginger in 1 liter of boiling water for 20 minutes. Drink 1 cup three times daily.

- Steep 2 teaspoons of rosemary 1 liter of boiling water for 7 minutes. Drink warm.
  Take 1 cup three times daily.

- Stir ¼ teaspoon of turmeric powder into a glass of warm water.
  Drink it twice daily.

- Steep 1oz of fenugreek in 1 liter of boiling water for 20 minutes.
  Drink 1 cup three times daily.

Health Tips

- Eat a well-balanced, healthy diet.

- Include lots of fiber in your diet.

- Consume coconut meat as part of your meal.

- Exercise daily for at least 30 minutes.

- Get quality sleep of 7 to 8 hours daily.

- If you have diabetes, try to keep it under control.

- Avoid smoking.

- Avoid alcohol consumption.

- Avoid coffee.

- Reduce your salt intake.

- Keep your blood cholesterol under control.

- Keep your blood pressure under control.

- Maintain your ideal weight.

- Reduce stress in your life.

STROKE

What is a Stroke?
A stroke is a sudden blockage or rupture of a blood vessel in the brain resulting in loss of consciousness, partial loss of movement or loss of speech.

There are 2 major types of Strokes:
Ischemic and Hemorrhagic.

Ischemic strokes are more common and are caused by a narrowing or blocking of arteries to the brain, resulting in severely reduced blood flow.

Hemorrhagic strokes are less common and are caused by bleeding in the brain.

Some of the causes are:-
Arteriosclerosis, diabetes, hypertension and tobacco.

Risk factors are:-
Age 55 or older.
High blood pressure.
Smoking, diabetes.
Heart disease.
Atrial fibrillation and blood disorders.
Migraines with aura.
Visual disturbances.
Family history.

Some of the symptoms are:-
Slurred or loss of speech.
Loss of memory.
Blurred vision.
Numbness to the body part.
Unable to swallow normally.
Fainting, coma.

The most common warning signs of a stroke are:-
Trouble walking.
Loss of balance or coordination.
Trouble speaking and understanding others who are speaking.
Numbness in your arm, leg or face, especially on one side of the body.

Other possible signs and symptoms include:-
Trouble seeing in one or both eyes.
Dizziness and complete paralysis.
Sudden severe headache with no known cause.

NATURAL REMEDIES

- Put a pinch of cayenne pepper in the food or drink.

- Use turmeric in your cooking.

- Eat lots of vegetables, raw garlic and fruits.

- **Nutmeg Liniment:** Combine 5 bottles of green rubbing alcohol, ½ bottle of white vinegar, 5 grated nutmegs and

2 tablespoons alkali. Bottle and rest for one week.
Massage the affected area every night just before going to bed.
N.B. After massaging with it, stay indoors and avoid going into water.

- Rinse the mouth with baking soda for thrush and bacteria.

- **If in pain** massage the area with cayenne tincture.

    Cayenne Tincture: Put 1 teaspoon of cayenne pepper in a glass jar, pour in 1 cup of rubbing alcohol. Cover the jar and swirl daily for three weeks then pour up the alcohol and discard the pepper.
    Apply to the area 6 times daily for 6 days, after that twice daily as needed for pain.

- **If not in pain** massage the area with 2oz of wintergreen oil mixed with 8oz of rubbing alcohol or coconut oil.

- Add ½ teaspoon of cayenne powder to a hot water bath.
  Soak in it for at least 20 minutes.

- Apply a fomentation to the chest twice daily if congested.
  Then massage.
  See the section on Hydrotherapy Treatments.

- A hot foot bath if not a diabetic.
  See the section on Hydrotherapy Treatments.

- Have a full body massage weekly.

Health Tips

- Eat a healthy diet rich in a variety of fruits, vegetables and whole grains.

- Consume coconut meat as part of your meal.

- Get lots of fresh air daily.

- Get at least 20 minutes of sunshine daily.

- Walk for at least 45 minutes daily outdoors.

- Do deep breathing exercises daily.

- Maintain a healthy weight.

- Avoid dairy products and meat.

- Avoid salt and white sugar.

- Avoid alcoholic drinks and coffee.

- Avoid fatty foods.

HYDROTHERAPY TREATMENTS

FOMENTATIONS

HERBAL TEA FOMENTATION:

1. Make an infusion or decoction.

2. Dip a towel folded in 2 or 3 layers the size of the body area you want to cover in the solution.

3. Wring out the excess liquid. Apply it to the affected area of the body.

4. Place a thick towel over the fomentation to help retain the heat longer.

5. Keep the tea hot and change the cloths every 3 minutes. Do 5 rounds.

6. End with a cold towel rub to the area.

HOT FOOT BATH

It is very good for headaches, colds, flu, coughs, congestion, nosebleed, earache, sinusitis, menstrual pains, fatigue, fever, pelvic cramps and congestion, prostate disorders, nervous tension, toothaches, backaches, infections, relaxation, stimulates circulation and warms the body.

Items needed:

1 bucket about quarter filled with hot water.
Small basin of ice water.
Large pan of very hot water.
2 washcloths for the head compress.
1 sheet and a blanket or 2 sheets.
1 hand towel for the neck.
1 bath towel.
1 bath mat.

Procedure:

1. Drape a blanket to completely cover a chair, then cover the blanket with a sheet.

2. Place a bucket ¼ filled with hot water on a bath mat in front of the chair.

3. Remove clothing, sit and wrap with the sheet, then the blanket.

4. Close all doors and windows.

5. Place the feet into the bucket and wrap the sheet and blanket around the bucket to avoid the circulation of air.

6. Wrap a hand towel around the neck to hold the sheet and blanket in place.

7. Apply a cold compress to the forehead, changing it every 3 minutes.

8. Maintain the water temperature in the bucket by adding more hot water continuously by pushing the persons feet to one side and
   placing your hands as a shield between the feet and the flow of hot water.

9. Continue adding the hot water for 20-30 minutes or an hour if needed. When sweating begins give the person water to drink at intervals throughout the treatment.

10. At the end of the treatment lift the feet up and pour cold water over them very quickly, dry and put on warm socks. Unwrap and dry the body. Dress, cover warmly and rest for 30-60 minutes. Take a cool shower.

A heating pad placed on the lower abdomen and upper thighs or a heating compress on the feet repeated every 4 hours can be used to replace the hot foot bath.
N.B. Do not use this treatment for persons with diabetes, loss of feelings, unconscious, arteriosclerosis, elevated pulse.

Other Book Titles by the Same Author

Can be viewed at this link:
http://www.amazon.com/author/monicasidoine

Home Remedies For Cancer

Home Remedies For Losing Weight

Home Remedies For Blood Pressure and Diabetes

Home Remedies For Headaches and Insomnia

Home Remedies For Sinusitis and Tonsillitis

Home Remedies For Constipation and Diarrhea

Home Remedies For Asthma and Bronchitis

Home Remedies For Dehydration and Vomiting

Home Remedies For Pneumonia and Tuberculosis

Home Remedies For Stress, Depression and Anxiety

NOTES

NOTES

NOTES

NOTES